Let's learn about "Power of Activity"

By Dr Jeremy Hawke (Podiatrist)

B. AppSc (Pod) M.A. (International Relations)

To my wife Jing and my daughter Qiqi, whose love and encouragement make this book possible

Contents

Introduction

Have you dreamed about opening that elusive door, where a higher quality of life awaits? Come and be guided. Where increased activity brings clearer vision, experiencing more vivacious colors. Where activity allows the sound of life to be celebrated. Life's scent becomes more intoxicating as your activity level rises. Your blood pumps in expectation of greater loads brought on by increased activity. Welcome to the power of activity. Here lies your chance to excel. Once you have mastered the power of activity, you will be the Genie who never returns to the bottle. Life has new layers. The new way of approaching life. Activity and the mind. How to harness brain power. Activity and the body with unlimited potential. Marriage of mind and body. Surprise yourself. Think about success in life. Boils down to your relationship with family and friends. The material stuff? Only a bonus for the journey of life. Improving those relationships that make up your success. An education. Life in new dimensions. You already have the motivation. Sustainability. Your internal genius. Your dream activities will mold you. Lower blood pressure. More muscle. A more sculptured body. Better intimate relationships. Change from within. Let us learn about "The power of Activity". Engage yourself in the benefits of increasing your activity level. Your body will never be the same and you will be shown how to get there.

By reading this book I will share lots of inspiration to keep you active for the rest of your life. Each chapter has step by step tips to help you stay on target, and reach your goals. There is a chapter on the different activity styles to choose from, and guidance on how to tailor a program for you. Examples include Tai Chi, Yoga, walking, Pilates and weight training. You will read real stories about people who have taken on the challenge, and turned their lives around. It is time to travel with me on a journey that may change your attitude to define health and activity. For instance, the low fat diet marketed in the United States in the 1970s hoped to solve the chronic disease problems of future generations. By cutting out fat in our diets, we have moved toward larger portions of low fat food, which often has thickening agents and emulsifiers added to make the food more palatable. Often these chemical compounds are fattening in isolation. This has led to more overweight or obese tendencies experienced by global societies. What we now have is a global epidemic of weight problems and over 66% of the global population considered as sedentary or inactive.

We are still being sold the concept of a minimum of 3-4 hours of medium intensity exercise as being required for acceptable fitness levels. People also think that a sedentary lifestyle during the day sitting down is fine, providing they are at the gym in the evening for their workout. Statistics are pointing in the direction of millions of deaths being reported, due to the long periods of sedentary behavior through the day, even with these exercise levels.

It is interesting to note that researchers around the world are now pointing towards consistent activity throughout the day, as being more influential on weight control and prevention of chronic disease. Recent research sites average fitness levels to be attainable by intense exercise for 3 minutes per week, under prescribed and monitored guidance. (Assessment by your medical practitioner as required). This indicates a whole new rethink of how we benefit from consistent activity right through the whole day. With average weight increases of 1kg per year in the general population, we have some noteworthy concerns about our future. So where do we go from here? Let the journey begin.

Chapter 1

The mind- Where the need for activity starts

Rising to your feet like a ringing bell,

Throughout your body sunlight shines,

Activity energizes each living cell,

A choir of life force making you move.

Fuelled by desire, you feel the excitement,

Cradled in the sumptuous lifting of spirit,

You are moving, yes moving!

Activity answered your highest prayer,

A gift of wise choices for you to share.

An explosion of joy, whatever you do,

Let no one judge, for the lucky one is you.

-Jeremy Hawke

Your exciting journey, transforming your health in so many positive ways. Up to 70% of most health problems will cure themselves. Mind directing the body. The other 30% will be in your conscious minds control. "Progress in motion". Harnessed benefits. Strong and sustainable health. Your relationship with the world around you. Longer life, better quality. Stronger muscles. Reducing weight becoming a reality. Improve bone density. Sugar levels in the blood clearing faster. Heart disease risk reduced. Less foggy mind but stronger postural muscles. Reduced risk of depression. Healthier circulation and increased flexibility.

Feeling connected and happy

Connectedness with society. You deserve to feel happy. When you are focused, decisions come easier. Lightness as you awake in the morning. Higher activity increases social integration, and depression is less likely.

Sally is 35, 168cm and weighed 90kg. On her initial visit with me, she was prescribed a 15 minute walk daily. Once her pain in the ankle had diminished through a set of podiatry treatments over a 2 month period, the walk was changed to 30 minutes and one Tai Chi class each week. Then in her workplace where she spent the whole day sitting at a desk, I advised her to stand for 50% of the time, and do the jobs standing up instead of sitting down. She now stands for returning calls. Two weeks later she had lost 1.5kg in weight, and sleeping better. She has better posture, less back pain and less fatigue, with more contentment and better intimate relationship with her husband and more communication with her children. After 6 months, her weight had dropped down to 78kg. She felt there's still more room to improve, but she was much happier. Sally feels "brand new".

Excitement, joy and happiness await. Making new friendships and social networks. The evidence presents positive outcomes for helping to lower depression levels. Much of the thinking relating to feeling fatigued and depressed can start diminishing. Hard to be depressed listening to classical music, isn't it? Imagination becomes creative, as you paint the activity on your personal canvas of life. So you will start to engage new ways of internal thinking about yourself, with less self-criticism. As you plan the new journey watch your internal genius becoming part of daily thinking.

Building the new brain map of your activity level

It is time for us to start building the new picture of what you consider your dream activity level. Start with a good design. The elements of a good design for higher activity. Purposeful application. Consider the following:

1. A reason for change.
2. A time to create change.
3. A building of persistence to stay with change.
4. A good diet to fuel the instrument-our human body.

5. A time to rest, when we have completed our activity.

6. A plan, so we have something concrete (but adaptable) to follow.

7. A mentor to help us understand the change we create, and not be overwhelmed by it.

8. A level of trust and faith in ourselves that these changes are positive and good for our lives, that we have a right to the change, which belongs to us.

Please take your time. Reflect on each point. Once you have done this think about your own personal activity level, and list your history of physical activity, sport, and work related activity level. You can do a past and present chart, so it is easier for us to work out how much more or how much less active you are now.It is only fair to start looking at some of the benefits that you, your family, friends and work colleges will start noticing:

1. You will take on a new confidence that people will notice about you. Increase activity levels will make you realize that you are capable of a lot more than you ever thought you were. This confidence will spill out into all areas of your daily life.

2. You will feel a lot stronger, and find that not only do you feel stronger, you actually are! This will lead to you being able to carry out a higher level of physical activity without getting so fatigued. Your energy level may rise, leading to a higher quality of life – "Work hard and play hard!"

3. You may feel a lot sexier. This is important to point out, because you are feeling more confident and stronger, you will feel and most likely be looking really good, and that will make you feel happier to be around other people that you want to be with. As social people it makes sense that we want to feel we are reaching our highest levels in this part of our life, no matter how senior we may be in age. Do not underestimate this point, it really does matter to all of us. We truly do care about how we come across to other people. And this is directly expressed in how sexy we feel, as this is metabolically controlled to some extent, and certainly neurophysiological controlled. Higher activity levels change our hormonal function.

4. You may feel a lot happier. Lack of activity often accompanies lack of involvement, which can lead to very negative perceptions about who we are and what we do. This can often lead to depression, which just makes things spiral in directions that we never intended to go in. Happiness is a state of mind, and often reflects the ability to see where we are going. Where we are going in life gives us all a sense of purpose and a sense of belonging in the big picture of life. Dare to achieve your human potential. One day at a time. Small changes add up to bigger ones in the overall scheme of your life. You may find yourself coming up with lots of new plans. You may want to change careers. Find a new partner for your new life direction. Travel to new countries. Earn more money or earn less money, in order to have more time for higher activity levels in your life.

5. Higher activity increases your intelligence. Exploring activity will introduce you to the science of neuroplasticity. This is one of the most crucially important and wonderful discoveries of modern neurology, that the brain in people of any age remains neuroplastic, and is able to continue building new pathways on a minute by minute basis for the rest of your life. How astounding is this? It has been known for a long time that we possibly only use a small percentage of our brains, the fact that you can increase your intelligence over time by developing new neural pathways is astounding. It will help you to make better decisions about your future, and what you want it to be.

"The secret of getting ahead is getting started".

-Agatha Christie

Chapter 2

The body-where activity changes your life

The sunlight bathed my soul as my heart beat rose

Another day of pure and unbridled activity

As I walk my muscles sing in delight

My blood flows faster mending its passages

Delivering nutrition throughout my body

My life feels exciting and filled with joy

To know I am new in so many ways

And improving my health is all these days

Come dance with me because now I know

How to step by step in the finest style

-Jeremy Hawke

From the first breath taken, there is activity within the body. Increasing it will reduce the risk of developing chronic diseases. The quality of life increases. Activity is defined as moving, working or doing something, the state or quality of being active. In addition to this,

> Body benefits through higher activity levels:
> 1. Reduction in body weight.
> 2. Increased muscle strength.
> 3. Lower risk of eye damage
> 4. Lower risk of hearing damage
> 5. Lower risk of falling.
> 6. Lower risk of damage to bones.
> 7. Better posture.

exercise can help drive us back in the direction of better health, if we already have a health condition or early potential of developing chronic diseases. Research was carried out by the Baker IDI Heart and Diabetes Institute and the cancer Prevention Research center at the University of Queensland. It was done in partnership with Medibank Private, a major health insurance company in Australia. The study was commissioned by Medibank Private and named "Stand up Australia". The statistics indicate the level of sedentary behavior that takes place in the areas of retail, call center and office based employees. 77% of the time at work for the study group, was spent sitting. These employees spent similar amounts of time sitting when having their time off work. Most of this group, only 5% of the day was spent doing moderate to vigorous level physical activity, and only 18% of the day doing light intensity (incidental) activity.

The research illustrates how widespread high levels of inactivity can be.

> *Recommended changes in your life style that complement the power of activity include:*
> 1. *Giving up smoking.*
> 2. *Cutting down on eating certain food that is not conducive to an active lifestyle.*
> 3. *Cutting down on your alcohol intake.*
> 4. *Sleeping earlier and wake up fresher.*
> 5. *Cutting out certain activities that create stress in your life.*
> 6. *Refraining from relationships with people who do not respect your long term goals.*
> 7. *Changing a job or start training for a new career.*
> 8. *Get a weekly or monthly massage to help reduce stress.*
> 9. *Buy a new wardrobe of clothes that go with your active lifestyle.*
> 10. *Join new clubs that allow you to share common activity and exercise goals, while making new friends at the same time.*

Any increase in your activity level leads to rewards. As you shift your activity levels your chance of a longer, happier and higher quality life increase. And the list goes on. But pay careful attention to the list above. As you honor the true you, your path to happiness is more defined.

Joan was a 45 year old lady who moved to Cairns two years ago. She had been working in a factory that preserved fruit in Northern Victoria. From a family of six children she had never known how to put herself first. She had been a mother of two children from a young age, and really needed to work full time. Her weight and work hours increased. Her lifestyle was inactive, she sat for 10 hours a day at work, and too tired to exercise after work. She felt depressed. She was overweight and suffered from lower back & knee pain. She did not sleeping well, and had no real hobbies. Work had become too painful for her, and she had been unemployed for 12 months. After we designed a podiatry medicine program to lower her pain levels, she applied the principles of the power of activity, and then watched her life change. 6 months later she had found a job in a department store, which really increased her activity level. Her mood lifted dramatically and she signed up for a local tennis club, an activity she loved when she was younger. Joan returned 12 months later, looking strong, lean and very happy. She said that the power of activity lifestyle had changed her ideas about her expectations in life. She feels that her life is so much happier now.

So harness the power of activity, and remember Joan. She had no idea what was in store. As you harness change, you will constantly surprise not only yourself, but the people you love in life. Once you start demanding to put ourselves first, things start to change. You will view every day in a new way. When you wake in the morning, it will be with a new view of life.

Diet and activity levels

A balanced diet is very important if you are going to increase your activity. The new food pyramid of healthy eating is a popular model for good eating habits, and puts more vegetables and fruit at the bottom of the pyramid, where we can eat more of this type of food, followed by grains on the next level. The third level includes moderate amounts of milk, yoghurt, cheese and alternatives, lean meat, poultry, fish, eggs, nuts and seeds. Healthy fats in small quantities are at the top of the pyramid. You can enjoy herbs and spices and choose water to drink. Salt and sugars are to be limited in use.

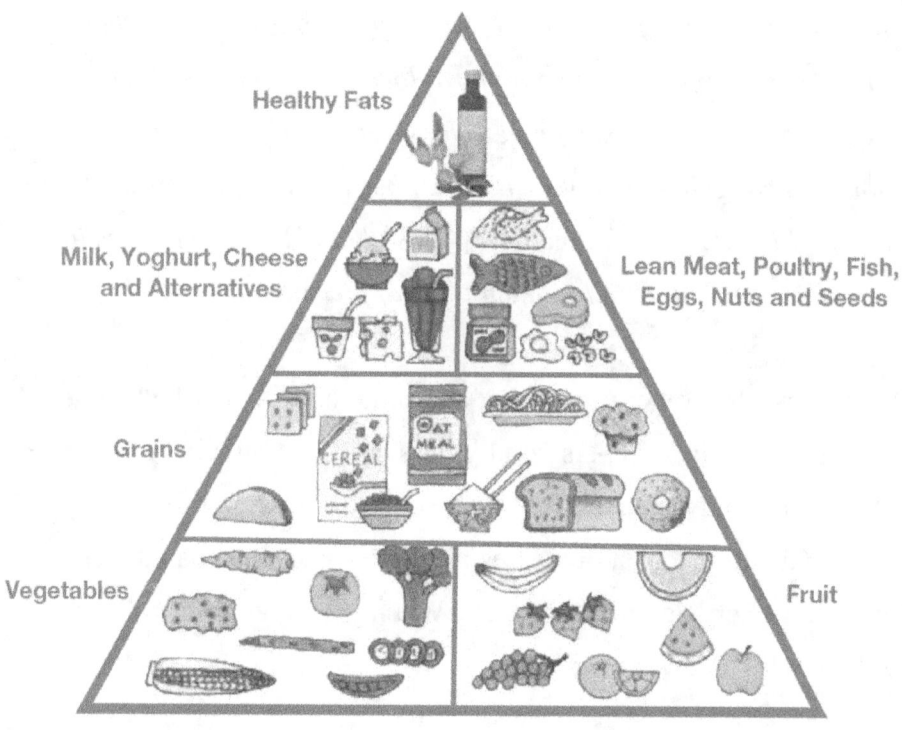

Nutrition Australian recommend a healthy balanced diet. This helps to avoid diet related diseases. Junk food should be avoided, and so should sugary drinks, see www.nutritionaustralia.org for further information.

Finding a balance in daily intake is vital. But you should also consider recent research into fats as an important consideration. Diet should always be considered in terms of energy consumption and energy expenditure. There have been studies demonstrating the link between the risk of obesity and inactive behavior. One of the best ways of avoiding this danger or moving away from the state of obesity, is by beginning a more active lifestyle. Manual farm workers in some countries burn up to 2400 calories per day, compared to 1200 calories per day for someone standing on their feet all day, and as mentioned earlier only 300 calories to be sedentary. These figures underline the importance in energy expenditure, when related to calorie intake.

There has recently been reports about the growing concern over previously help perceptions about the negative aspects of having fat in our diets, in the mid-1970s large amounts of money were spent on research into the benefits of low fat diets. Because of the enormous cost of the research, bit money was spent marketing these low fat eating habits in the western world. What was being ignored was research only soon after the release of the low fat diet research, indicating that fat was an important part of our diets, and helped in some ways to wash out the arteries and other blood vessels, and turn our appetites off when we feel that we have had enough to eat. We must therefore exercise constraint with fat content of food, but not cut it out totally. Same goes for carbohydrates, the brain needs them, and therefore there should be a balanced intake of them. Consult a Dietician for specialist advice on dietary concern.

"Take care of your body. It is the only place you have to live".

-Jim Rohn

Chapter 3

Mind and body -

The roadmap of how to become more active

I am myself, I am always here.

I am you and you are me.

Make me active and I will grow,

but sit me down and we start again.

When will I be active?

Guide me and nurture me, love is for the best.

I will sleep for rest.

Till then I will dance, stand, jump and prance.

Surprise me and use me,

Let's see the world.

-Jeremy Hawke

This is a model to bring together more information to help you analyze the direction you will be travelling in on our activity journey. It is just amazing how much our own personal records of our activity levels can help us to be pushed further forward towards reaching our full potential. Remember that the information you are collecting can be added to by you. Anytime you like. Start by drawing up a chart like the following one I am demonstrating here, with lines and columns to enter the following information each day.

1. Number of hours slept and quality of sleep, either poor, fair, good or sublime.

2. Pulse rate. (Check glossary for further details)

3. What you had for breakfast, lunch and dinner

4. What snacks you had, including alcohol consumption.

5. How much water you drank during the day.

6. How much exercise you did including type, intensity and duration.

7. What your activity level was, including hours spent and type.

8. How you are generally feeling, including physical and emotionally.

9. How you feel today about your future activity levels, i.e. optimistic or lacking confidence.

10. What your weight is and how you feel about your body image.

Here is a list of the things that are now becoming part of your daily experience:

1. *A better understanding of the benefits associated with higher activity.*
2. *A better understanding of how to incorporate these changes into your life.*
3. *An understanding of the brains capacity for change.*
4. *A realization that through neuroplasticity changes, you can really change the direction and appreciation of your higher activity levels.*
5. *A more positive outlook on where you are now, and the direction you are heading in with your increase in activity.*
6. *A better appreciation of the high value of activity other than exercising in a general sense.*
7. *More belief in your own potential to internally tap your own personal genius.*

There are many electrical devices, like Fitbit and apps that will store some of this information.

Analysis

Now is to chart these variables into your chart over the next 3 months, daily. Start now! This will save you from thinking in three months "Wow, how did I get to this point"? It will also allow you to assess the performance of that wonderful piece of machinery - the human body. Just like the McLaren racing car or champion team athlete, it requires careful performance analysis to see where progress lies, on a day to day basis. This information inspires you to watch your own progress. The aim is for you to take total control and be the Captain of your own ship. It will allow you to measure your increased activity levels, and also measure what effect this is having on your sleep, diet, snacking, and the way you are feeling physically and emotionally. Do not worry if your weight is not changing much, your clothing may be getting looser even though your weight is not changing, as you may be putting more muscle weight on.

Your new roadmap of activity starts with a plan. First decide to dedicate some time. Always best to select what fits in best with work and home. Before the family gets up in the morning is good. Get honest. How many hours per day are just spent sitting? Take these hours and try this first. Every 20 minutes of sitting, follow with 2 minutes of gentle walking. The benefits through the day are listed in the Table blow.

Benefits of not sitting for long periods
- *Less internal inflammation*
- *Better blood sugar clearance from circulation.*
- *Better fat clearance from circulation*
- *Better stomach muscle strength*
- *Better back postural muscle strength*
- *Better hip flexor strength*
- *Less damage to the heart*
- *Less work for the pancreas.*
- *A clearer head.*
- *More calories burnt.*
- *Better muscle/fat balance over time.*

"It is not who you are that holds you back, it is who you think you are not."

-Unknown

Chapter 4

Power of activity and preparing your body

My life was in a state of sedation

My day was sedentary, foggy, unsure

I was shown a new path to expand my life

I stood up and kept standing and moving

Now my unhappiness is history, just a mystery

Once you really move, you choose to groove

You will never go back to Aladdin's lamp

You are as free as a bird, reaching high

No limitations ever again

-Jeremy Hawke

Prepare for physical activity increases. There are some important considerations. We come from a variety of backgrounds:

- You may be 45 years old and have not exercised for 20 years.
- You may be an elite athlete who had an injury two years ago and want to return to a higher level of activity.
- You may be a 20 or 30 year old embarking on a new exercise plan to be more fit and fashionable.
- You may be a teenager and want to join a new sports team with your friends.
- You may be a 55 year old who sustained an injury at work three months ago, and wants to get your fitness level up to go back to work.
- You may have type 2 diabetes and be 40kg over weight and need to introduce exercise as part of your Diabetes management.
- You may be a 10 to 12 year old who wants to increase their activity for a snow board competition or hip hop dancing.
- You may be senior and in danger of falling and need exercise for falls prevention.

Therefore we must share a starting point, let us divide activity into groups:

1. Sedentary activity level: Mainly refers to sitting or lying down.
2. Light intensity activity level: cooking, walking, hanging washing out, sitting at a computer, standing and reading a book.

3. Moderate activity level: Walking, fishing, water aerobics, mopping and vacuuming.
4. Vigorous activity level: Riding a stationary bike, using a rowing machine.
5. High intensity activity level, running over 15km/hour.

Daily requirements of moderate activity should be 40 minutes. Warming up and cooling down before exercise is important.

Good exercise programs include:
- *A level of intensity not exceeding our capabilities.*
- *A level of duration which meets our conditioning level.*
- *A rest period allowing intervals for recovery.*

Have an activity plan. Visualize yourself succeeding. Visualization allows you to see it. For instance, if you are going to imagine yourself running 500 meters, visualize tying up your shoes laces and standing up to prepare for your run. Imagine how the ground feels through your feet. Is it warm or cold? Listen to your breathing. Break into a gentle jog and feel the increased force of gravity affecting your relationship with the ground. Think about how you feel about this relationship with the earth that you are running on. Feel gratitude. You are now starting to think about your running through a process of mapping pictures in your mind that build a run into something like the real thing. It has also been demonstrated in some research that the mind does not necessarily know the difference between the real thing and visualizing the real thing. Interested? It can therefore be beneficial as preparation for different types of activity. In addition to this, it can be beneficial during times of injury, or rehabilitation from an injury.

There is a very famous Formula 1 racing car driver named Jackie Stewart, who discussed a race at the famous Monaco grand prix. He described how he could picture the race track in its entirety and know exactly what gear he was going to select for that corner, what line he would take through that corner, and what his physical relationship with the car was, depending on whether he was racing in the dry or wet. By the power of visualization he was able to practice racing his car, which has enormous sports medicine demands on his body and concentration. The use of highly sophisticated EEG equipment for measuring brain function can demonstrate that while Jackie was going through that process of visualization in his mind, he was actually using muscle firing pathways that would be firing the muscles required to carry out that activity of racing a formula one racing car.

Let us start with a walk

Walking is a remarkably good activity for building your fitness. No matter the distance you choose, you will end up being "walking fit". Start small and you can build up over time. If you are just walking you can adapt the intensity, duration and intervals of your walks at your leisure. Once you are fit enough to do this, you will always have a routine to come back to. If you already walk regularly or you just prefer to move into running, then by all means you can do this.

Checking your fitness levels

It is a good idea to make an appointment with your General practitioner or doctor before embarking on big increases in your activity level. As some of the suggestions I share with you will require either moderate or larger levels of exert, a medical clearance is a good idea. If you are looking at running, it may be wise to consider a stress ECG, to make sure that any potential cardiac issues are identified early. It is surprising what additional confidence you will have in developing sustainable increases in activity, if you know that you have been assessed as medically fit to do so. If the doctor has concerns about your fitness levels, there may be some modifications of these recommendations required, to better suit your level of fitness. This may include consideration of any additional medical conditions that you have.

Maintaining good levels of fluid hydration is essential as your intensity and duration of activity increase. Regular hydration with water helps prevent you from getting dehydrated. Consider using electrolyte replacement with water intake, as this helps with fluid absorption and electrolyte balance. Fatigue can sometimes be due to over training, and could also indicate that you may be getting dehydrated. Watch for both of these things. And remember, moderation is good in the early stages of training. This is not about a program to do for a month or two, this is about building sustainable activity into your life, and being able to maintain this in the medium to long term.

Warming up

A little routine that is simple and easy, that will warm up the muscles, ligaments and tendons, and help increase the blood circulation to these tissues. Warming up is a really good practice, which will help to prevent injury. As you are going through the following routine, you are gently stretching the tendons of the foot and lower limb, and you will gently apply forces to the insertion of the tendons and ligaments on the bone surfaces, signaling them to prepare to adapt to the loads you are planning to place on them. If you have been doing some of the visualization techniques recommended earlier, this may have also assisted in your preparation. In the colder months of the year, it is recommended to warm up for a little longer. In the warmer months, do not neglect at least the minimum time devoted to warming up. Funnily enough, you will more than likely end up enjoying this time. Up until about the age of 20 years old it is easier to think that warming up is not necessary, and you may well get away with ignoring it. But as each decade passes after reaching 20, the elastic quality of our soft tissues starts to reduce, and we are for this reason more prone to injury while increasing our activity levels or exercising. So just see it as an investment into the future as you increase your activity.

First warm up sequence

You can sit yourself down on the lounge with your feet in front of you, flat on the floor. Now gently lift the heel off the ground as you rise up into the ball of your foot , and then gently lower down. Repeat this eight times. Follow this with lifting your toes off the ground with the heel staying on the ground , and repeat this eight times too. Now lift the foot sideways, causing the big toe side of the foot to lift off the ground , and the little toe side of the foot to stay on the ground. Doing this with both feet four times, and then reverse this, so the little toe side of the foot is lifted off the ground , repeat this four times as well. (A little harder). Now turn to the left side as you lie one leg along the lounge with a straight knee , and gently lean towards the foot , which will warm up your hamstring. Reverse this sequence for the other hamstring (hold 8 seconds each leg). Once you have done this, go back to the sitting position and lift the right knee up, so the foot lifts about 50cm from the ground, and repeat this four times for each knee, which will warm up your hips. Lastly, place your feet under one knee at a time, and hold your one knee with both hands while you use your big toe to draw the alphabet, using the whole range of motion of your ankle as you carry this out. It can be in upper case, lower case, Chinese, English, Italian or any other language you like! But this alphabet sequence is a gem, as it confuses the firing order of the muscles so the brain does not know what sequence of muscle use is coming up. It is very good to warm up all of the lower limb muscles. Now you can stand up, and do a simple squat at Thai Qi speed, that is very slow as you bend your knees, and very slow as you stretch your knees. Around 4-6 slow squats and you are all ready to go. The lovely thing about this simple sequence is that it prepares the lower limb architecture in both its anatomy and physiology state, and allows you to safely increase your following activity levels over the next one hour to one and a half hours. This is starting to get exciting!

The warm up sequence described above can be helpful for many reasons. It will allow the bones, muscles, ligaments and tendons to be slowly prepared for higher levels of activity. Even though it is a simple routine, you can add to it over time, depending on your own personal requirements. Keep routines simple. It helps to develop consistency.

Preparing your gear for your walk

It is important to have well-fitting comfortable clothing for your walking. It should be brightly colored if you are walking at night. You do not want the clothing to be too tight or too loose. A zip pocket in your shorts or track suit pants is handy for carrying a key. Be careful not to carry multiple keys in your pocket when walking in groups, as other walkers may find it very distracting to listen to rattling keys. Your T-shirt may be short sleeved or singlet type. Socks are also very important as you do not want the socks to bunch up in your walking shoes, or to have seams which cause discomfort to the feet. Some walking socks are marked left and right, to help ward off blistering of the feet. This can be very effective for some people. It is helpful to have two or more sets of clothing for your walking. You do not want to be discouraged from walking just because the walking gear is in the wash. Pick good quality gear. It does not have to be very expensive, but look around before you buy, and try the gear on.

Shoes

One of the most important pieces of your walking apparel will be your walking shoes. The important point here is that walking shoes vary greatly in quality. The good news is that you do not need to spend a fortune to get a nice pair of walking shoes. The important thing is to decide on your budget for shoes. Remember walking is for everybody. Do not feel your shoes have to be expensive to start with. The things you will be looking for should include the following:

1. The shoes should have a good non slip sole that has an appropriate tread for the surface you are walking on.
2. Lace up shoes are best, Velcro may be suitable for people who have trouble tying laces.
3. They should fit well. Allow your own thumb to be put in front of the big toe, allowing your foot to lengthen as you walk.
4. The lighter the shoe the better, but it must still fit well.
5. Try and have a good shoe fitting technician to help you fit the shoe. Some specialist sports shops can be good for helping you with this very important point.
6. The shoes should allow for good ventilation while walking, to help dissipate perspiration.

Picking your surfaces to walk on

This is nearly as important as a good walking shoe. Early in your walking career a softer surface may be beneficial to help prevent injuries. Bitumen and concrete are examples of surfaces with little or no give in them, so they offer no shock absorption. Walking can generate considerable amounts of force. On a surface with no give, this may put more strain on your body. If you pick walking on grass instead, this will lower the force on your feet and lower limbs. Be careful in parks and on tracks, where small to large holes may be obscured by grass or undergrowth, and you could easily have your foot fall in the hole and injure yourself. One of the best surfaces for beginner walkers, is that wonderful modern day invention, the treadmill. Do not be put off by people stories about how boring it is walking on a treadmill. We are trying to guide you to sustainable increases in activity. There is plenty of time to get out and pound the pavements safely and injury free, when your feet and lower limbs are ready.

"A fit healthy body - that is the best fashion statement".

-Jess C. Scott

Chapter 5

Power of Activity and planning for success

My thoughts dance like beautiful music,

painting a dream of great majesty;

the drums beat fiercely bringing focus,

my heart feels great excitement;

new plans begin to bloom,

and connect me to visualization

of my fantastic new equation.

-Jeremy Hawke

Your plan will allow you to be on target, for the rest of your life. The rewards that you attain will belong to you. Nothing left to chance. Measure your progress in motion. It is about devising strategies to be a winner. To start enjoying the benefits, a record of how you got there. Remember our discussions regarding a daily journal? This is always an important part of planning for success. Our daily activities do not always leave time to remember everything. So a journal allows us to remain connected with our long

Your new daily experience:
A better understanding of the daily benefits.
A better understanding of creating change.
A better appreciation of higher activity.
A more positive outlook.
A better appreciation of the value of activity.

term success.

Always remember the words of the leader Winston Churchill, "Never, never, never give up". Far too many people give up when

they are just about reaching the point of success that they desired. Whether it is just to become a more active or become a world leading athlete, the possibilities are equally viable. You know when you hear people say "Oh well, we will see what happens"? It leads to you being controlled by circumstance, and most people allow this to happen. Chronic disease takes place over time. An example is chronic heart failure, which can affect a significant population of people over the age of 50 years old.

Here is a project for you. Let us prescribe an increase in activity for you that you may not have at the moment. Stand up for 15 minutes of each hour you normally spend sitting. This is a new level of advancement from your 2 minute walk every 20 minutes. Keep the 2 minute change in place. If you normally sit for eight hours a day, it would look like this. 2 hours more of activity. Plus the addition of your 2 minute walks. Multiply this by 7 days and you have 14 more hours per week of activity. This is an important start, as you readdress the belief about what it means to be active. So often you can be discouraged from taking up physical activity because you think that 40 minutes of high impact activity is the only way to get fit. Again, try and move away from this being the only possibility. It is more important to be doing small amounts of activity right through the day. As mentioned earlier, when you are up and standing, your body is able to clear out more blood sugars from the circulation per hour, leading to less internal inflammation and less risk of development of chronic disease from this inflammatory phenomenon.

Rest is also an important part of the new direction you are heading in. Keeping the strategies simple is really important. Once you are heading in the direction of more activity, you will be surprised how much fatigue and mild depression will diminish. You become part of the creative process. And when you start designing your increased levels of activity, negative feelings will start to be replaced with a new sense of excitement about where you are going. Life is not about where you are, but more about where you are going. You will be developing new ideas about your activity levels. As you develop new ways of thinking about an active life, you may then wish to teach these things to your children or grandchildren. And who knows, they may go to school and discuss it at show and tell, or teach it to their friends. And here lies our opportunity to integrate our teachings into the lives of our dearest children and grandchildren.

Remember, it is within your control to decide exactly where you would like to be in 20 years' time, activity wise. What weight would you like to be? By doing some planning together, we can select the basic ingredients of the activities that are part of your life. Until you make a plan, you will not find the inspiration to be totally committed to all of life's possibilities. Isn't it empowering to know you can really have anything you want?

There can be distractions that can pull you away from the activity level you desire. So rather than procrastinating about activity levels, let's work on it now. Find a balance between those activities that appeal to you. Write it down. Start that routine. Starting a new routine is a good opportunity to consider the program design. When you are designing your program, it is a good time to decide what you actually intend to get out of it. Do you want to be stronger? Would you like to have more stamina? Do you want to improve your balance? It is very interesting when we start asking these questions as it allows us to pick the most relevant activities.

"Days of my own making pass sublimely, for through my dreams I believe all is possible".

-Jeremy Hawke

Chapter 6

The investment into posture and breathing

Your activity bank is always open,

From the moment you become awoken.

If we know our reason to toil,

Then never will our body spoil.

For the lessons we learn right now,

Are ingrained in our minds, anyhow.

-Jeremy Hawke

It is difficult to face some simple facts of life. We came into life with no guarantees of success or failure. We know higher activity levels are reported to be good for us, but rarely do we see how we fit into this big picture. We are linked in many beautiful ways to our friends and family. But rarely do we stop to consider what this means. What does it mean to be linked by love to them? In more than one way it means having a social responsibility towards these people. This is where our perspective of higher activity levels needs to change.

To feel gratitude towards the changes taking place in your life is crucial. Seeing good health as something secondary to our existence makes no sense at all. How often do we find ourselves pushing for deadlines, and ignoring our own wellbeing? If we do this, we are not having gratitude for the opportunity to enjoy the highest possible level of health and fitness. The homeostasis within our body relies on us consciously getting some things right. As we do not want to head in this direction, we must acknowledge the rewards that we will most likely get.

- An increased sense of self-worth.
- A happier and healthier friend, parent, spouse, son, daughter, sibling or co-worker.
- An increased excitement for living life rather than just feeling like an observer of life.
- A feeling of belonging in a healthy active society.
- New networks and friends who enjoy our chosen path as much as we do.

- More money in our back pocket due to health increases.
- Less missed days from work.
- Less chances of developing diabetes.
- More stable blood sugar levels in the presence of diabetes.
- A more stable blood pressure.
- Potential improvements in blood pressure if we have been hypertensive.
- A lower chance of developing further blood vessel disease in the form of Atherosclerosis.
- Less chance of heart attacks.
- Less chance of becoming overweight or obese.
- Chances of stabilizing our weight if we are overweight or obese.
- Lowered chances of developing some cancers by reducing risk factors related to sedentary behavior.
- Improved intimate relationships.
- Improved chance of forming intimate relationships.

Some essentials for high activity levels

There is a small toolkit of things which are essential to sustaining high levels of activity. I will cover these briefly to give you some guidelines how to achieve these things in your toolkit. The first one to consider is posture.

Posture

Good posture is required, in order to stand, walk, run and carry out many other activities. What do we mean by good posture? In order to carry out the activities listed above, we need to be able to balance when we walk, and maintain a skeletal position that allows us the best chance of carrying our body. Good posture is important, as we are less likely to injure ourselves and will expend less energy carrying out daily activities, if we pay attention to our posture. Let us look at some of the attributes of good posture that you can start working on. A well trained dancer is a good starting point to study posture. Look at a classical ballet trained dancer and you will see some interesting things. Their shoulders are open but not pulled back, and there is no slumping forward. If you look at the neck position, it is as if somebody has attached a piece of string to the top of their head and pulled it up. The neck is beautifully lengthened. Now look at their ribcage. The stomach has been gently pulled in and they have lifted up underneath their diaphragm, and have taken care not to arch the back when doing so. Now observe the pelvis. It has not been pushed too far up, but it has not been allowed to slump forward. The balanced position of the pelvis allows for a very naturally straight back position. Now look at the legs. The feet are not too far apart, just about hip width apart and the feet in a relaxed but not too far turned out angulation.

Now I would like you to attempt the same position. Putting your back against a wall and gently bending your knees will give you a feeling where the back should be. Now that you have tried this new postural position, I want you to work on it for the next 6 weeks until you own it. Until it excites you, and makes you feel stronger throughout the day and more prepared for all the increases in activity that you are going to be involved in. Over the next 6 weeks, you will not only feel better, but you will even look better. When you walk you will enter rooms commanding attention. Your organs will be less stressed because you are supporting them better with your muscles and skeleton. You do not have to be a professional athlete to get the benefits of a superb posture. You may also find that you are getting less back pain. When the posture is allowed to slump, the strain on the lower lumbar vertebrae is increased significantly. You may also find you are breathing better. Again, bad posture does not allow the lungs to function as effectively, so now you will be able to take air in without so much strain on the lungs.

I recently had a patient come and see me who had been having a lot of lower back pain, which had led to her decreasing her activity level significantly, for over 2 years. Her shoulders were slumped over when she sat in the chair. Her weight increased by 10kg over the two year period, and she was feeling depressed. After two sessions of working on her posture, she went away and worked on the recommendations I had made, and returned to see me 6 weeks later. She walked into the room with a beaming smile and sat down with a really good posture. She told me that she had not felt so good for many years, and she had lost 2kg of weight, as she had been able to return to a 30 minute daily walk. She was feeling much happier, and I asked her to come back and see me in 6 months.

This is one of many hundreds of stories that gives you an example of the power of good posture. Our modern lifestyles of sitting in front of computers and slouching over desks, has led to a reduction in opportunities to work on good posture. And it is not something that we ever get much tuition in while we are growing up. But good posture is important. Never underestimate the potential of small alterations in posture influencing our lives. As you integrate postural improvement with your increased daily activity, you will surprise yourself. Your vitality levels will start lifting and you will feel more youthful. You will find people noticing something different about you, but not necessarily being able to put their finger on what. But the important thing will be how you feel inside as a person.

I encourage you to work on posture for your children/grandchildren. They are also getting less opportunity to work on good posture. Observing them at the dinner table is a great place to start. But again it is necessary that good posture extends into all parts of their lives.

Breathing

Breathing is an important part of increasing your activity level. Awareness of breathing during activity can be very important in supporting good activity. There is a very important link between the quality of breathing and posture. When we are pushing the lungs during high levels of physical activity, the lungs are capable of carrying up to 100 liters of air supply, to take oxygen to our muscles to allow us to move. What we tend to believe is breathing is just a part of everyday physiological function. True. What we are referring to here is improving your breathing in order to gain the health benefits from correct breathing. When you are maintaining good posture in both sitting and standing positions, the lungs are able to draw air in more freely during inspiration. The inspiration phase of breathing allows the alveoli throughout the lung to receive the required oxygen. These are little sacks that receive oxygen and prepare for its transport to the blood coming from the heart. Here the blood receives fresh oxygen that attaches to the hemoglobin in the red blood cell and goes back to the heart to prepare for being pumped throughout the body. Do you think the amount of oxygen going to your body is important? The answer is yes. There are a lot of benefits to breathing in a more efficient way. Breathing is tied up with some of the most vitally important functions of our brain. The nervous system is divided into the central nervous system and the peripheral nervous system. Both of these systems are directly linked to our breathing, some by hormones called acetylcholine, which are chemical neurotransmitters that control parts of our nervous system. I will talk about them in later books in more detail. Now to talk a little about the expiration or exhaling of air from your lungs. Back to the alveoli in the lungs. These are the clever little sacs we agreed pick up the fresh oxygen for our body. But in equal importance they are dropping off the carbon dioxide from around your body, the waste product of our Krebs cycle, the wonderful cycle that makes energy production possible in our body. So what is happening? Our improved posture is starting to let us get rid of the waste products in our respiration, all that carbon dioxide that needs to be released through expiration or breathing out. Is this starting to get you a little excited? I think perhaps it is! Our body is the most brilliantly designed entity that you could possibly ever imagine. All of the muscles and soft tissues that allow our lungs to breathe are just magnificent. And here is the most inspiring part, you have control over these lungs, and you can guide them and pilot them by your increased level of activity. You can therefore assist in helping your nervous system to function better. Some of the advantages of breathing better will be listed:

1. It can assist in leading to you being more relaxed, which can be beneficial to helping to regulate a better blood pressure.
2. It will allow better distribution of oxygen throughout your body and improve the health of the tissues of the body.
3. Your increase in activity will move you away from the feeling of short of breath, and the normal feeling of breathlessness while exercising.
4. Activity increase will lead to less oxygen being needed for allowing muscles to move, and less production of carbon dioxide by the muscles.

If increases in activity level lead to fatigue, coughing or shortness of breath, you should see your doctor as soon as possible to see if any further lung examination or testing is necessary.

Chapter 7

Activity and our health

My days are now enriched by wealth,

As I build by health with leisurely stealth.

For now I realize I did not know,

What health and activity daily show,

In knowledge that the difference,

My heart will know.

-Jeremy Hawke

There are some changes in your daily health that are demonstrated quickly. Our body benefits in many ways, following activity increase. Immediate changes in blood flow quality and quantity. Higher levels of oxygen transported throughout our systems. Growth of new cells to build structures to take on new tissue loads. Have a look now at what changes are taking place in your bones and heart, one vital system supporting your body and the other pumping blood.

Bone health

Increasing your activity level is a vital ingredient to maintain good bone health. Weight bearing activity is the best for maintaining good bone density. You should be doing at least regular moderate intensity exercise to strengthen up your bones. There are some interesting things to remember about bone density. Up until approximately 31 years of age, we are depositing calcium into the bones by a process known as calcium banking. If you can imagine your bones being a bank that you are depositing calcium into up until this age, it is a good way of looking at it. After this age the bones start having calcium leeched out of them, and maintaining weight bearing activity becomes vitally important to maintain bone density. Bones are fascinating. Not only do they support us, but they provide new red blood cell production for our circulatory system. (More oxygen carrying cells remember?). Growth factors and cytokines are manufactured in our bones, and it also acts as a calcium reservoir for calcium homeostasis throughout our bodies. (For instance, muscles need calcium as part of muscle contraction). Bones are made up of both cortical and trabecular bone, with a protective layer called the periosteum. The periosteum is a fibrous protective layer of the bone. I have some wonderful news for you. Moderate level weight bearing exercise improves the quality of the periosteum layer of the bones, which means the more you are doing this type of exercise (i.e. brisk walking) the better the quality of the periosteum layer of the bone. This means more protection for the bones. The vital components for maintaining bone density must both be attended to for maximum bone strength. Firstly you need a sufficient intake of calcium, which needs to be in the presence of vitamin D to allow the best absorption of calcium. Secondly you require adequate and regular weight bearing activity in the presence of the calcium intake, in order to maintain maximum bone density. This is a crucially important reason to support increased activity levels. It is a vital one to remind our children, grandchildren and parents about. The long term dangers of not paying attention to bone density maintenance is Osteoporosis. Osteoporosis is a bone disease where there is insufficient calcium deposits in the structure of the bone, to maintain sufficient strength in the bone. If this condition exhausts, it can lead to a greater danger of the bone breaking. People with osteoporosis should be very careful about exercise involving bending forward, or activities related to bending forward. Discussion with your general practitioner or physiotherapist is wise, to help design special exercise programs when Osteoporosis is present. Bones are in a constant condition of change, they are being built up and broken down on a second by second basis, allowing older bone with micro damage to be repaired and replaced. It is worth noting here as I can hear some of you asking. Does Osteoporosis affect the ability of a bone to heal if it is broken? The answer is not always. The ability of the bone to heal itself is not always affected, but the danger of having fractures present are more than often related to the bed rest that may be required while for instance, a hip or femur fracture repairs. The dangers can include deep vein thrombosis and other circulatory dangers, that in themselves can be life threatening. So we must never underestimate the incredibly important place that activity has in promoting bone health.

Heart health

Activity increases will lead to much better heart health. There are many important blood vessels throughout the heart that are involved in transporting blood around your body. Far too often, people are not alerted to the dangers of heart disease, until the heart fails. The heart is a massively strong muscular pump, which is capable of pumping up to four times as much blood around your body while you are exercising.

Some of the benefits of exercise for the heart include:

1. Lowering the risk of getting heart disease in the future.
2. In the presence of coronary heart disease, exercise can lower the chance of further heart attack or reduce the dangers of further

heart disease. It can also help to protect your heart with the presence of coronary heart disease.

3. Exercise helps to protect your heart as well as improve high blood pressure, Diabetes and high cholesterol levels.
4. Increased physical activity is good for people who have had heart attacks or heart surgery.
5. Many other types of heart conditions are helped by regular physical activity.

It has been widely reported that up to 70% of women and 60% of men in the U.K. do not get enough exercise to protect themselves from coronary heart disease. Similar statistics are present in Australia. It makes you realize how important it is to address sedentary behavior, where one out of five cases of heart disease takes place in developing countries, for this reason. If you have high blood pressure you should discuss what types of exercise to avoid. It has been demonstrated in research that moderate level intensity exercise on a regular basis, can help you to prevent developing high blood pressure. In people with high blood pressure, 30 minutes of moderate intensity exercise on a daily basis can help to control high blood pressure, which in turn will help the heart to function better and lower the risk of heart attacks and strokes.

Sam, a 42 year old was referred to me by his medical practitioner. He was 120kg, and had a history of high blood pressure and had been diagnosed as being pre diabetic. After examination and assessment I started him on a walking program which brought his weight down to 100kg. After consultation with his doctor, I recommend a running program. He commenced running 3km three times a week and joined a running club. He has now ran his 8th marathon, covering distances of 42.5km. He cannot ever remember such high fitness levels in his life. He is now socially active in his running club, and is looking at going overseas to run in the London marathon. When he first came to see me, he would have had trouble running for a bus. His life has changed through the power of activity. His blood pressure is close to the same as someone half his age. His blood sugar levels indicate a reduced danger of Type 2 diabetes, and his weight is down to 80kg. He does not feel lethargic anymore, and would love to still be running marathons at 80 years of age. I told him that should not be a problem, there are many people running marathons at that age.

"If we could give every individual the right amount of nourishment and exercise, not too little and not too much, we would have found the safest way to health."

-Hippocrates

Chapter 8

How much and what mix?

There is an answer in your heart,

That surely wants to make you start,

To create a trail that you will know,

Will lift you skyward through energy flow!

-Jeremy Hawke

The following recommendations will give you a guide to how much exercise should be blended in with your other increases in physical activity levels, to lead to getting the benefits of increased health. Firstly, approximately 150 minutes of moderate intensity exercise should be in your weekly plan. How do you know the activity is moderate intensity? You should notice your body is warmer, your respiration and heartbeat rise, and then you can still carry out a conversation while exercising. In addition to your 150 minutes of this type of activity, you should also do some muscle strengthening exercise. This can be done by lifting light to heavy weights, and advice from your doctor should be sought if you have any medical conditions. If you are over 65 years of age, you should also be doing work for your balance for falls prevention.

Safety

Just to mention a few points on safety again. It is important to choose activities that allow them to be carried out with an acceptable level of safety. This becomes more important in senior years, where discretion and further guidance may be needed before embarking on certain activities. Do not be afraid to stick to a very basic exercise and activity plan. Having regular variety can help to prevent you from becoming bored with your program, and not continuing it. Take care with activities like swimming if you have any heart conditions. While it can be very good for some heart conditions, it may not be good for others. It is therefore best to ask your doctor or cardiac specialist for further guidance. Some activities where holding the breath and straining (i.e. weight lifting) may not be good if you have high blood pressure, as it can push the blood pressure up even higher. Correct guidance should be sought from your doctor in this situation, as alterations in your training techniques may be required. Remember to be flexible with your mix of activity. There is no harm in trying a particular activity for a while, and changing to another one if you need to.

"You only live once, but if you do it right, once is enough."

-Mae West

Types of activity mix.

Low level intensity activities.
1. *Slow walking.*
2. *Standing and carrying out activities like ironing or reading or bird watching.*
3. *Standing cooking, small cleaning chores.*

Types of moderate level activity
1. *Certain types of housework, including brisk mopping,*
2. *Brisk walking.*
3. *Dancing classes.*
4. *Swimming.*
5. *Aerobics.*
6. *Climbing stairs.*

Strength building activity.
- *These activities can include digging in the garden, using resistance style bands, lifting and carrying shopping, climbing stairs, lifting light and heavier weights at the gym. Tai Chi and Pilates.*

Balance activities.
- *Activities for improving balance include cycling, bowls, Tai Chi, Ballroom or line dancing, and classes specifically designed for falls prevention exercise.*

Chapter 9

Power of Activity to develop our social networks

Through activity let us find a friend,

For in our growth we truly mend,

All those cells that surely grow,

With vitality and kindness, yes we know.

-Jeremy Hawke

There is an extremely satisfying aspect of increasing our activity levels. It is the connections with people in our lives. Since the industrial revolution, opportunities to network have steadily slipped away. Circumstance compounds this:

During a period of illness.

Following rehabilitation for an injury.

Following retirement from a career.

Following loss of a spouse.

Following a period of depression.

Following the birth of a baby.

Following loss of contact with social groups when looking after ageing relatives.

Many people feel very much like you. They may have the same level of fear about going out and meeting new people in a group they have never been to. Once you have been to a few meetings of activity groups, you will slowly become more familiar with the people around you. You will also be meeting with a group of people who share a common belief, that they believe activity is important in their life. Secondly, there are so many different types of activity related networks that you may be able to join. These can include walking clubs, cycling clubs, Tai Chi clubs, running clubs, numerous sporting clubs for different sports, dancing clubs, falls prevention groups, and so on. The opportunity to network with other people has many advantages. It allows you to share your passion for activity. It can lead to long term friendships with people who will help motivate you to stay with your new found activity levels. It can even lead to activity levels increasing in a much safer environment, which can help to further encourage your ongoing involvement. So have a think now about what activities you may enjoy. Are there any activities you did when you were younger, that perhaps you may like to return to?

Grace is approaching her 80th year of age and had been noticing unsteadiness in her walking. She had a hip replacement 12 months ago, but the pain had not reduced much. This led to 11 to 12 hours of sitting during the day. Her back was aching and she was feeling very foggy in the head. I designed a Podiatric medicine treatment program for her hip pain, and then prepared to build her strength and confidence up again. I asked her to start with a two minute walk every 20 minutes throughout the day, for each hour she was just sitting. After my recommendation of a free council Tai Chi class and a falls prevention course, she started attending them both once per week. Three months later she reports that she is sleeping well now, with a marked improvement in her appetite. She no longer has hip pain and feels really clear in the head. I am now starting her on a brain exercise program to help improve her special awareness for preventing danger, and her memory and navigation skills. This will help her not only to better identify danger, but will give her more confidence when out navigating new locations she visits, on her new journey of activity. She has made some new friends and reunited a long lost friendship she had from 3rd grade at school. She reports that she never knew how happy it was possible to be at her age, as she enthusiastically waits for her 80th birthday. The new activity level Grace has started will build new blood vessels in her limbs for better blood transportation. As she adapts to the new activity level, she is helping to maintain her calcium deposition in her bones, keep her muscles strong and assist in preventing further falls. Her heart will remain stronger, with better clearing of blood sugar and circulating fats throughout her circulatory system.

"Success is getting what you want, happiness is wanting what you get."

-W. P. Kinsella

Chapter 10

Activity for children and grandchildren

Don't wait for tomorrow to live,

Life is not a dress rehearsal.

Work is only work until it is fun,

Activity will nourish as you run.

Don't be frightened by what you achieve,

Activity is your future, no need to grieve.

Be happy, I will show you the way.

Get active, the world is your stage,

Dance like no one watching,

While you sing of lives great joy.

-Jeremy Hawke

There is clear understanding that children's young mind is highly

influenced by actions and directions surrounding them. There has
been a concerning shift in the activity levels of children, to the point
of actually being able to call many children's lifestyle sedentary.
Adult lifestyles have become hugely dependent on cars. For all the
wonders of modern technology, we have been persuaded by clever
marketing that more of these cars are required. So children are also
affected by these changes. With limited time, it is easier to jump
into the car to get from one place to another, running to a tight
schedule of course! Telling the children not to worry about walking
to the local shopping center, easier to drive them there, it will save
the time. Not only easier, but safer. The concept of safety for
children and grandchildren is based on concerns about their safety,
mostly based on experiences about the danger surrounding them and
also rightly or wrongly, by media reports. Add to this cocktail the
time some children spend playing electronic games, being on
Facebook or YouTube, sitting doing their assignments on the
computer. Letting children go out and play on the street is becoming
a thing of the past, and through these and many other examples,
children and grandchildren are leading more sedentary lifestyles.

It is necessary to step aside in many ways, to ensure that the needs of
the children are put absolutely first. If you are a Parent, you know
this better than anyone. Parents will sacrifice just about anything, out
of love for their children and making a safe, excellent and
sustainable future for them. So here is the frog sitting in the water

that grows slightly warmer every day, and the frog does not notice any difference. But if the water continues to get too warm for them, they may perish without ever knowing why. Look at the evidence. Children being overweight and obese is rising at alarming rates. Children as young as 10 years old are now getting high cholesterol levels, heart disease, and high blood pressure, and increasing their likelihood of having a higher risk of developing cancer and Type 2 diabetes.

If change is to take place, let it take place on a micro level, and let it expand from our local communities. Change can come from within. Governments can help change the direction, but you can take a horse to drink the water, but you cannot make the horse drink that water. The horse needs to want to drink the water. And the ways of doing this include the following:

1. Leading by example.
2. Integrate our teachings about becoming more active and share it with our children.
3. Children can be rewarded for changing sedentary behavior.
4. Encourage them to follow healthy role models.
5. Being there for them if all of the above fail occasionally.

6. Trying not to judge, but to support.

Some activity suggestions with your children include:

- *Taking up a sport with your children that can be shared through the years. As they say, families that play together stay together.*
- *Organizing bush walks or walking tours for your children and their friends.*
- *Encouraging children to get up and walk for 2 minutes every 20 minutes, so they start to think about getting up and doing more active things for themselves.*
- *Suggesting some physical activity that must come before they are allowed to start sitting and watching television or playing computer games, Facebook, etc.*
- *Arranging desk heights for your children which will allow them to stand while they work on a school assignment or do their Math and English exercises.*
- *Go for an early morning or evening walk with your children.*

Influencing our children's activity levels

Leading by example is probably one of the most important aims. Every parent in their heart will try and do their share of guiding, nurturing, keeping safe, loving and supporting their children. But sometimes there is limited time. It comes back to community. The important thing to remember is that change is happening around you at a rapid rate. So the next extension of this influence can be increasing personal activity levels as leaders for our children, and doing more activity related things and exercise with them. It is like forming an own personal micro-government, and appointing parents/grandparents as the leader of the activity department. Write the new policies for the department. Have faith that it can work. Another advantage of starting children moving towards these habits, is that they will be inspired to teach their children the same things when they have their own children.

Stewart is in his early thirties and was looking for some changes to his activity level that would allow him to involve his family. I advised him to consider some walking along the local Cairns Esplanade with his wife and children, rather than the family sitting at home in the afternoon watching television. Stewart returned to see me a month later to share his story with me. The whole family was loving the new quality activity, and they're inventing things to do after their 3km walk. One week they took a Frisbee to the park and threw it for half an hour after the walk. The following week they took a basketball and shot hoops. Now it had become a competition to come up with the best activity after walking. This has led to over one hour per week of extra activity with improved quality of health, more family time, and opportunity for new activities. Stewart and his wife have decided to buy some bikes for the family and integrate riding into some of their trips.

"The pursuit of truth and beauty is a sphere of activity which we are permitted to remain children all our lives."

-Albert Einstein

Chapter 11

Power of Activity for Falls prevention

I have known your voice, touch, smell and taste since birth.

Your cradling support in my first moments, my bond absolute.

Your guidance created familiar from unknown, splendor from mystery,

My memories of our divine history.

Your independence marks strong defiance,

On ever being seen to indicate reliance.

Success we measure in the relationship we treasure,

Caring for you being my great pleasure.

-Jeremy Hawke

There is a strong link between higher activity and the incidence of less of falls. Research demonstrates a great cost to society from falling. The risk of falling can take place in many situations, including the workplace, out in public, and at home.

Benefits of activity for preventing falls:
1. Improved balance from higher activity.
2. Better concentration when walking.
3. Better recovery from close falls.
4. Better workplace, public place and home safety.
5. Less risk for missed time at work.
6. Less chance of injury or hospitalization.

Returning to activity after inactive periods

It is best to start slowly after periods of inactivity. You may have a memory of what a high activity level is like, but your muscles are probably not conditioned to take on too much load. It is advised to start with small challenges and then build them to a higher level. Reasons for periods of inactivity may include: Illness, rehabilitation following an accident, or declining levels of activity taking place with age. You must remain positive about the direction you are aiming in. Try very hard to be focused. It often helps to write a set of goals down on a piece of paper or in a journal.

Start small. Daily walks of 15 minutes would be a good start. Housework counts as activity, do half an hour of housework and write this in the achievements area. Add standing time too, perhaps 15 minutes out of each hour you spend sitting. A good place to start. By achieving this on a regular basis, you will get a good basic level of strength going. Building up from here is not too difficult. You may like to get a personal trainer to assist you for two half hour workouts per week, if you feel the need.

Increased activity following an accident or an operation

Very often guidance by a health professional will be required for an initial period of post-accident or post-operative rehabilitation. But very often the programs only go for a short period of time, and you are left with a certain number of guidelines telling you what you cannot do, but very little about what you can do. Lying in bed for extended periods of time can lead to muscle strength losses of up to 1.2% per day. You need to regain your strength, to return to the same level of functioning that you had before an operation or an accident. Be careful not to fall during these periods of time. Once your muscle strength decreases, your ability to walk properly is often severely reduced. In situations where you could very easily catch yourself if you kicked uneven ground or stepped off a curb, it may not be possible in these circumstances.

Strategies to help reduce falls

1. Enroll in a falls prevention class (Where required, and is worth serious consideration for all people over the age of 60 with a falls history).

2. Take extra care after long periods of being confined to bed. Not only are your muscles not as strong, but proprioceptors throughout your lower limbs and feet are not functioning correctly. These proprioceptors assist in telling your brain where you are in time and space, every time you stand or walk. They are helping to provide information in the form of sensory nerve reposes, to help adjust your balance. When they are not fine-tuned by regular practice, your chance of falling is much higher.

3. If you have had any medication changes or changes in medicine dosage that make you feel dizzy, speak to your doctor immediately. Feeling dizzy is not normal, and if medicines have led to this dizziness, you will be in greater danger of falling. This type of problem is more common if you are on a large number of medicines.

4. Have a look at active thinking and consider walking and Tai chi as part of your activity plan.

5. Now for something very important in relation to increased activity after sedentary periods. Staying out of danger of falling requires concentration. Do not let your concentration be distracted while walking. If an emergency takes place such as

kicking an uneven pavement, our concentration cannot take us from our thinking in the form of a distraction, back to the emergency. We may be lying on the ground after falling, looking up at the crowd around us, before we realize what just took place.

"Age is no barrier. It is a limitation you put on your mind."

-Jackie Joyner Kersee

Chapter 12

Power of Activity and building our confidence

Procrastinating can affect our activity levels and our motivation levels. Try to be kind to yourself on days where you are not sure whether you feel like being active. Sometimes you just run out of time. Does this mean that you have lost our routine? No. The beauty of setting a routine is that you have one. There are many ways of dealing with these type of days, but there are a few guidelines to handle interruptions.

Be kind to yourself, be proud of how far you have come. It takes a master painter a long time to paint a masterpiece. You are no different. Take time to create your masterpiece of activity. The benefits are going to travel with you for the rest of your life.

Missed days are statistically small percentage wise compared to the number of days in the year that you will not be missing. Take confidence in that fact. So if you miss a day occasionally, enjoy the rest.

Speaking of rest. Sometimes a low confidence day may be just because you are tired. Learn to listen to your body. When you need to rest, create the environment to rest. Take some time out. Get together with a friend. Take a trip to the art gallery. Get well hydrated. Check you are eating properly. Watch a favorite movie or read a book.

It is better not to force higher activity when you do not feel like it, or just do not have the necessary time to do the activity. Remember, you are human. If you are not feeling like being active, consider looking at some new activities to keep you interested and fresh.

Have you overbooked your day? Sometimes expectations are set too high. Often this is setting ourselves up for failure. So beware of the danger in over commitment. Unfortunately we equate high achievement with others approval.

Confidence levels

Confidence levels take time to build. You will observe increased familiarity expectations you have placed on yourself. Changing them can be confronting. Doubts creep in like "do I really have time for this? Or "shouldn't I be devoting this time to the welfare of my family" and so on. Not giving ourselves enough private time can lead to these types of feelings. Confidence relating to physical activity levels may be low if there was little regard for physical pursuits when you were younger. Research demonstrates that if we keep heading in the direction of inactive behavior for another 10 years, 80 percent of the world total population will be overweight.

The good news is that you do not need to be part of this statistic. Why not settle for an increase in activity levels and a sensible well balanced diet, and be prepared to enjoy the journey of losing weight over an extended period of time? Dieticians will most likely agree. Our activity levels and diets need to be balanced. Everything in life has a natural balance and homeostasis. Activity should be fun. It should bring you joy. As you get stronger and healthier, feel the excitement and joy from your achievements. And the beautiful thing is they are not going to go away. You will learn to master the techniques of self-management. How empowering is that?

Fatigue

Just a few more points about fatigue. Fatigue is a very important symptom that may be trying to tell you something. It may indicate an illness or more likely be symptomatic of our low levels of fitness. If you are feeling fatigued and not noticing these levels of fatigue dropping, it may be time to see your local general practitioner and have a medical checkup. It can also be related to over training, and not having enough intervals in between our activity program, to let our body recover. These tend to be common symptoms in professional athletes and dancers and shift workers, where they are not having time for their natural homeostatic balance to be taking care of things, and allowing them to wake fresh from sleep to face another busy day.

Body image and activity

Body image is a sensitive subject. We all want to look our best. Most of us also think that we should look even better than we do. This is not an unusual feeling. There are many reasons why carrying extra weight around can be very troubling to us. Within our profession research demonstrates that the population is getting one kilogram heavier per year as adults. Look around and you will see both at schools and society in general, we are getting bigger. Often a person will look at another person and say to themselves "I am glad I am not that big". Society does pass judgement. There seems to be many reasons for this, and they are often unfair and illogical judgements. They may be related to religious teachings of size relating to gluttony being one of the seven deadly sins, or if there are so many starving people around the world, why are people getting so big? This is where body image can often make one shy about increasing our activity levels in public or exercising around other people. If this is a reason for you having trouble sticking to a program of increased activity, be kind to yourself. Try your hardest not to look back into history to find the answers. Take one day at a time, remember and realize as your confidence levels grow, these feelings will slowly start to reduce. Do not ever, ever, ever give up. You may be closer to your success than you ever know.

Ethnicity

We are a culturally diverse planet. The planet is made up of many different ethnic groups that live side by side. It is a duty to mankind to work together as a team, to make sure that there are equal access to resources, whether they be food, shelter, education, health or technology. In order to work together and raise our planet to its highest capabilities morally, spiritually and economically, we must encourage equal access to these commodities as humanly possible. So if there are any reasons that you feel unable to reach your highest levels of activity related to the subject of ethnicity, then it is time for change. Society must work together and grow fitter and healthier together. Things that we must all teach our children, that equal access is a necessity, otherwise it would be unjust. And no more unjust than to ourselves, if we are denying access to activity for these reasons. We must always fight any tendency that we have, to shy away from integrating ourselves into access to physical activity and health. If you feel this way, you must discuss it with friends, family or a health professional. Life is to be lived, and you must allow yourself and be allowed to express yourself without judgement or discrimination. Our humanity is a shared humanity, excision of anybody for any of the reasons above cannot be tolerated, ever.

Peer pressure

So often people who love activity in their lives, are surrounded by family and friends who tell them to grow up and stop trying to behave like a twenty year old. You may have questions aimed at you like: Isn't that what young people do? Why would you bother wanting to do all that activity, what difference is it going to make to your life? But here is the real deal. This is your life. What you decide to do is based on what you think the best. The truth is far more different than this. It is fun. It is good for you. How much you decide to do is entirely up to you, and what you plan for in activity increases will reap rewards accordingly. Once your peers observe the progress of your activity level, they may very well be following your footsteps.

"If you always put limits on everything you do, physical or anything else, it will spread into your work and into your life. There are no limits. There are only plateaus, and you must not stay there, you must go beyond them."

-Bruce Lee

Chapter 13

Making activity choices that interest us

Let us go out for some activity today,

And work our frustrations into play,

No doubt our choice will reflect,

The dreams we are yet to perfect.

Do not wait another day,

For activity is coming your way!

-Jeremy Hawke

Aim at making your own blend of activities that you feel comfortable with. Now it's time to look at a short list of some activities I think you would enjoy. There is also a short discussion on the merits of some of these activities.

Walking

Walking is one of the best ways of increasing your activity levels, without putting strain on your body. One of the most appealing

aspects of walking is that you can literally do it anywhere that you like. By changing the places that you walk you can lower the chance of getting bored and losing interest in the activity. All you need is a pair of walking shoes and you can be on your way. You can choose the level of intensity from a gentle walk up to a much higher intensity walk.

Swimming

Swimming is a very relaxing activity that can also be varied in

intensity. By using different swimming strokes you can enjoy a variety of strength and stamina improving exercise. Do not be discouraged if you are not a strong swimmer. With some regular tuition you are able to build some basic skills which will heighten your enjoyment of the activity. As swimming is non weight bearing. It is very good to do if you are injured or senior in age. There are also some wonderful group activities that can be done in the water. The first one that comes to mind is water aerobics. Even if you are not a strong swimmer, you can do a class that is carried out in shallow water. These classes can be absolutely fantastic if you are looking for a non-weight bearing form of exercise. Often if you are recovering from an accident or operation, water activities can be excellent. Another highly underrated activity in the water is water walking. By wearing a weight belt around your waist, you can walk from shallow to slightly deeper water, and get some non-weight bearing or semi-weight bearing walking in. This type of activity is also great if you are suffering from arthritis or lower body pain that makes exercise more difficult otherwise. For the more adventurous, swimming squads and water polo can be a lot of fun, and are often tailored to different levels of skill and fitness.

Cycling

Cycling is a very good activity for raising your fitness level and also allowing you to relax at the same time. It gives you a choice between cycling outside or being on a stationary bike and carrying out the

activity at home or at a gym. It can be a light intensity right up to high intensity activity, which allows you to adjust it to your own requirements. When you start a cycling plan, remember to start your training gradually. Your back, hips, knees and ankles all need time to adapt to the new level of activity. It is also important to have a bike properly set up for you, in order to get the best out of your riding. It will not only allow you to perform better, but also help to stop you from getting injured. Bikes do not have to be ultra-expensive, but they need to be designed well. If you are riding an outdoors bike, always protect your head with an approved helmet. It is really the only safe way to ride. Some countries do not require you to wear a helmet. Believe me when I say you need to protect your brain. It is vitally important to prevent head injuries as much as we possibly can.

Tai Chi

Tai Chi is an activity that is first carried out in groups with a teacher, but as you learn some routines can be then carried out by yourself. You are then able to do the routines at home or in a park or perhaps on the beach. Not only is this activity very good for your fitness, but it can be extremely good for lowering your stress levels.

You could regard it as a form of meditation in motion. There are some excellent evidence based studies on the place of Tai Chi in falls prevention. This can be a superb activity. One in three people over the age of 65 have a fall each year. It is therefore a very good activity for seniors, and will help you to build your lower limb and upper body strength, while relaxing at the same time. Often local councils will run these classes, which you can attend free of charge or for a small fee.

Yoga

Yoga can be a wonderful form of exercise, and like Tai chi, it is considered to be meditation in motion. More advanced forms of yoga require extremely high levels of skill, so they have to be approached with great respect and care, and always under the guidance of a highly skilled and qualified teacher. Not all yoga has to be practiced at such a high level, but you are more likely to stick with it if you are attending a class. At least when you just start.

Weight lifting

Weight lifting is an immensely valuable addition to increasing your activity levels. It has been long believed to have limited benefit to your cardiac health. This has now been disproven,

Lifting light to heavy weights is actually having a profoundly good effect on your cardiac health. It is a superb activity to start changing the balance between fat tissue and muscle tissue in the body. It also happens to largely influence the laying down of new bone tissue, allowing ongoing improvements to bone density. Adding between one and three sessions of weight lifting can be an excellent addition to your weekly activity levels. I recommend consultation with gymnasium staff or a personal trainer for guidance. Good technique is important for weight training. Weight lifting can also assist in preventing injuries that may present in other sports. It is also helpful for preventing falls.

Fitness Trampolines

Fitness trampolines are very good ways to boost your activity. They do not take up much room, and can be excellent for indoor activity when space is limited. There are different routines you can carry out, and you may be pleasantly surprised how well a fitness trampoline fits into your routine. They are capable of giving you an aerobic workout, while strengthening your gluteal and limb muscles. It is a low impact activity, and can burn approximately

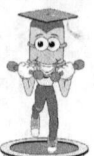

180 calories in half an hour.

Pilate's classes

Pilate's classes are designed to work your whole body, in machine based and non-machine based styles of working out. The Pilates system was originally designed to assist professional dancers with their strength and injury prevention. These classes are very good for building core internal muscle strength and can be especially good in rehabilitation from injuries. It is best to consult a

professional Pilate's teacher, who will be able to ensure safe, progressive and sustainable benefits from this fine pursuit.

Activity variety

I think you can comfortably say that there are so many variations in the numbers of activities that you can choose from. Once your confidence level grow and you believe that you can do anything that you want to, you become very empowered by this knowledge. Being empowered leads to having more choice in your life. This is the pivotal point where you see the advantages of increased activity spilling into all areas of your life. To give you an example, you may find yourself surrounded by new offers and invitations to engage your company, in situations that you never would have entertained in the past. And so these are the changes we put in place, without even realizing that these changes in your life are taking place, your whole world is changing with hundreds of millions of new connections taking place in your brain structure. Up until now you may have experienced little changes taking place over weeks and months, as your activity levels changed. But what you are actually doing is inventing a brand new you. Do not be overwhelmed by this thought. As time goes by you will be surprised how your taste changes, and you become more confident at making new choices that suit you most. This is natural. It does not mean that you do not have the discipline to stick with a small number of activities. It may just mean that you are wishing to be challenged by new possibilities. That is a wonderful thing.

Chapter 14

Conclusion

Bringing the power of Activity together

Often there are times in life where change makes a rainbow of new possibilities seem logical. Very often the first step in a new journey. It is only in reflection we see where change came from. All of a sudden higher activity levels do not seem to feel so foreign. Your progress is reflected in your determination. You have come so far in such a short period of time. Here is an exercise for you. Can you make a list of the changes that you have carried out so far? Now next to each change list the benefits you feel you have made by implementing these changes. If you have just read the book through from start to finish, list the changes you would like to make, and what you believe the benefits will be. I recommend keeping this book by your bedside, and you can read sections of the book again as you choose.

The beauty of life will shine even brighter for you from now on. You are unlocking many parts of your own brain that will be preparing you for further changes in your life. You have to keep on dreaming. Remember not to be frightened away from the things that you truly desire in life. By following the guidelines in this book you have started to prepare your life for anything that comes along. So choose carefully in all areas of your life. Do not be scared to dream big. No matter what you aspire to become in your life, you can have it if you believe that you can. If you believe, then you must carefully plan how you are going to go about getting what you desire. The more value of what you aspire to, the more diligent you will have to be to follow it through. Do not ever give up on anything you want or desire, because the genius inside you deserves whatever you believe you deserve. It will all come back to you. Decide to take responsibility to carry out all the work that is required to achieve your success. Remember to be patient, for success comes to those who are patient. And patience therefore requires perseverance. Sometimes you may have a quieter period of activity, and if you do, enjoy the rest. Luxuriate in your rest. Spoil yourself. When you are ready to go back to your higher activity level, guess what? That fantastic routine that you have so masterfully built with the assistance of some guidance from this book, is going to be waiting for you.

So remember, it is a big world. But there is only one of you. You are unique. You are so, so, important. You are beautiful. You are strong. You are kind and compassionate. You are understanding. You are caring. You have a responsibility to the family and friends that love you so much. Share these teachings with those you love. Because we are one family, one giant family who are on a spiritual journey together. We need each other and must bring the best out in each other. You deserve the best. Your body truly is the temple you thought it was. You must prepare this temple with gentleness and kindness and tolerance. Be kind to yourself. Do not punish yourself. If some of the concepts take a little while to get working together with your busy life, do not worry. Just pat yourself on the back and be patient. Success after all should be based on your relationship with your friends and your family. Everything else in life is just a bonus. So let your increase in activity make that relationship with all those you so deeply love, even healthier, happier, and more prosperous. May we all travel together through our lives as happy as we can be? We are travelling together. Can you feel it? Sure you can. I can, you can be sure of that.

One of the good things about this book, is you can return to read it, as many times as you like. Each time you return, I believe your higher activity level will continue to remind you, as these pages do, about the power of activity. Have a great active day!

"I've missed more than 900 shots in my career. I've lost almost 300 games. Twenty six times I've been trusted to take the game winning shot and missed. I've failed over and over and over again in my life. And that is why I succeed".

-Michael Jordan

Jeremy Hawke 2015

Exams for the power of activity

The following exam is to test your knowledge on the power of activity. Please feel free to repeat the exam at a later date. You may find this helpful to test your understanding of the subject. Select true or false for your answer to the following questions.

Q1. Visualization for activities you may practice or plan to practice, can be assisted and even improved by this process.

Q2. The recommended break from inactivity is 2 minutes each 20 minutes, which will help to prevent long term chronic disease.

Q3. Variety will not help prevent boredom in your activity program, it will just make things complicated.

Q4. It is never too late to change your activity levels, quality of life can be enjoyed at any age.

Q5. It does not matter if your children see you as being inactive, they are probably paying no attention.

Q6. Falls prevention programs can increase your safety and attention to potential danger.

Q7. The brain cannot change as you grow older, so there is no need to bother trying.

Q8. Body image cannot change, it is something you are born with.

Q9. Increasing your confidence with activity can lead to new opportunities in many areas of life.

Q10. Increased activity levels throughout the day cannot make any difference to your health.

Q11. Good breathing control can help you with gaining better health long term.

Q12. Heart health has nothing to do with activity, it is just about pumping blood.

Glossary

Balance

Balance is a biomechanical process where the center of gravity is able to be maintained without too much postural sway. It is made possible by complex changes in muscle firing and relaxing, and the input from proprioceptors, which measure your position in time and space when standing. These systems are controlled by the central nervous system. It involves vestibular, somatosensory and visual systems for continuous monitoring and control of balance.

Blood pressure

Blood pressure is the pressure of the blood that is travelling through the blood vessels of the body, and is worked out by multiplying the heart rate by the peripheral resistance. Blood pressure is measured by taking a systolic and diastolic measurement.

Cognitive

Cognitive refers to the set of mental abilities including memory, attention, intelligence, evaluation, reasoning and judgement, that allows us to process information in order to make decisions throughout our daily life, based on our gathering of knowledge and experience.

Falls prevention

Falls prevention becomes more important as we age. The danger of having falls increases due to many factors, such as decreased cognitive function, reduced sight, muscle weakness, medications that are prescribed and non-prescribed, dangers around the house and community that may lead to tripping and changes in height of suffices, slipping in water, or not seeing steps. There are many good programs for seniors in the way of falls prevention courses, which can be extremely valuable to lower the risk of falling. Contacting your local council or doctor would be good sources for more information on these services.

Homeostasis

Homeostasis is the continual monitoring within a system to allow a stable and constant state within a particular system.

Neuroplasticity

Neuroplasticity refers to the ability of our nervous systems to change over time. This involves changes in both neural pathways and synapses, and can lead to us learning new ways of processing information. This can include navigation, memory, intelligence, memory, fascial recognition, speed at carrying out particular activities, and emotional changes. Increasing activity levels can potentially lead to changes taking place in some or all of these areas of neurophysiological function. Neuroplasticity change can have a profound effect on neurological functioning, leading to very large changes in our lives. Areas that show special promise are recovery from brain damage, learning, and cortical remapping after injury. It is also known as brain plasticity.

Pulse rate

Pulse rate is the number of beats the heart is making, often measured in beats per minute.

Exam answers

Question 1 True

Question 2 True

Question 3 False

Question 4 True

Question 5 False

Question 6 True

Question 7 False

Question 8 False

Question 9 True

Question 10 False

Question 11 True

Question 12 False

Acknowledgements

I would like to acknowledge the diligent research carried out by the scientists in the field covered by the material in this book. I thank them for it. Without their sincere and compassionate research, less progress in preventing chronic disease would be made. Great thanks to my wife Jing for her tireless editing, formatting & publishing of my work, which would not have been possible without her. Thanks to Tony for his illustrations and book cover work.

References

Alkhajah TA, Reeves MM et al. Sit-stand workstations: a pilot intervention to reduce office sitting time." Am J Prev Med 2012 3(3): 298-303.

Thiorp,Alicia, Dunstan, D; Clark, B.; Gardiner, P.;Healey, G.; Keegel,T.;Owen,N.; Winkler, E. Stand up Australia. In collaboration with Medibank Private. August, 2009.
Armstrong T, Bauman A, Davies J. Physical activity patterns of Australian adults. Results of the 1999 National Physical Activity Survey. Canberra, Australia: Australian Institute of Health and Welfare; 2000.

Chau JY, van der Ploeg HP et al. A tool for measuring workers' sitting time by domain: the Workforce Sitting Questionnaire. British Journal of Sports Medicine 2011 45(15): 1216-1222.

Commonwealth Department of Health and Aged Care. National Physical Activity Guidelines for Australians: Active Australia. Canberra, Australia: Commonwealth Department of Health and Aged Care; 1999.

Dunstan DW, Salmon J, Owen N, Armstrong T, Zimmet PZ, Welborn TA, Cameron AJ, Dwyer T, Jolley D, Shaw JE.

Associations of TV viewing and physical activity with the metabolic syndrome in Australian adults. Diabetologia. 2005; 48:2254-2261.

Gorman E, Ashe MC et al. Does an 'activity-permissive' workplace change office workers' sitting and activity time? PLoS One 2013 8(10): e76723.

Hu FB, Leitzmann MF, Stampfer MJ, Colditz GA, Willett WC, Rimm EB. Physical activity and television watching in relation to risk for type 2 diabetes mellitus in men. Arch Intern Med. 2001; 161:1542-1548.

Owen, N., Bauman, A. and Brown, W. (2009). Too much sitting: a novel and important predictor of chronic disease risk? British Journal of Sports Medicine, 43, 81-83.

Pugh, C.J.A., Sprung, V.S., Ono, K., Spence, A.L., Thijssen, D.H.J., Carter, H.H., Green, D.J. 2015, **'The effect of water immersion during exercise on cerebral blood flow'**, Medicine and Science in Sports and Exercise, 47, 2, pp. 299-306

Salmon J, Ball K et al. Outcomes of a group-randomized trial to prevent excess weight gain, reduce screen behaviors and promote physical activity in 10-year-old children: switch-play. Int J Obes (Lond) 2008 32(4): 601-612.

Thiorp,Alicia, Dunstan, D; Clark, B.; Gardiner, P.;Healey, G.; Keegel,T.;Owen,N.; Winkler, E. Stand up Australia. In collaboration with Medibank Private. August, 2009.

Nutrition Australia
www.nutritionaustralia.org/national/resource/healthy-living-pyramid

www.ingramcontent.com/pod-product-compliance
Lightning Source LLC
Chambersburg PA
CBHW062013280526
45787CB00005B/2090